A Message from Apostle

How do God create something new through you? By first creating something new in you. Once healing is visualized, the evidence is internalized, it will not be a surprise that by his stripes we are healed.

In May of 2020 God charged me to go on a seven day fast. I started the fast, at the end of 7 days the Lord visited me and told me that this fast had to be 49 days. I followed the Lords instructions but had no idea that I was about to embark upon a journey that would change my wife and I lives forever.

As I begin the second week of 7 days our bodies begin to be riddled with pains day to day. We spent countless days in the E.R. and Minor Medicals in between the first 8-21st days of this fast.

After the rounds of E.R. visits we experienced a severe Achilles rupture that required emergency surgery and the rest is history. I remembered that a year to date of this surgery I was hospitalized for a life-threatening illness. As I am thinking on the illness and the surgery the Lord begins to tell me his plan.

The Lord tells me that he is releasing something new in the earth through our ministry. This is a new dispensation of healing. He then tells me the reason I had to fast for 49 days. The Lord stated that this was Prophetic symbolism of testing and completeness.

Therefore, as you go on this healing journey with us. The Lord will heal your body, mind, and soul as he had healed us during this time. At the end of the fast I had fully recovered from a surgery that should have taken at least 6 months to be walking. Every ailment that had troubled us was gone. Healing is released in Seven times seven it is time to take up your bed and walk.

~Apostle J. Lamon Brodnax

Forward

Apostle J. Lamon Brodnax is a true God's man. I know him to be a servant leader, godly role model for his children and the flock that God has assigned him to. He is very humble, compassionate, and trustworthy.

During the 2020 COVID-19 pandemic, God commissioned Apostle Brodnax to go on a journey that he was not familiar with. God charged Apostle Brodnax to fast for seven days, then God turned it into forty-nine days. In the mist of him accepting the commission, various things begin to come against his body as well as mine. I can remember going back and forth to Campbell's Clinic to see what was going on with him as well as myself. Pain begin to consume us, and we did not have a clue of what was going on or why this was happening. The more we prayed and fast, the more our joints began to afflict this pain upon us that we had never felt before.

I believe it was June of 2020, Apostle Brodnax and one of his associates decided to co-host a session and scripture free play social event for the community. Everything was going well, and everyone was having a great time and suddenly, something happened. Apostle Brodnax went up to score two points, but when he came down, there was a loud sound to come from his ankle. Out of all the years that Apostle have lived, he never broke a bone in his body but the moment he decides to honor this great commission that God commission him with, things started to happen to his body. He ruptured his achilleas, and because he went to the ER during a time that a virus consumed the world, they didn't see a rupture but only a sprain. It was not until he went to Campbell's Clinic that he knew the severity of his ankle. Surgery was needed immediately according to the doctor and it was to the doctor's surprise that Apostle Brodnax was still walking on his ankle.

Can I tell you that during this forty-nine days of fasting afflictions came over Apostle's body. Can I tell you that though they came, God allowed healing to take place in his body in a super natural way: mentally, physically and emotionally. It is my belief, that God allowed Apostle to undergo various afflictions in his body to produce healing. Not just for him but for those that's currently connected to him and for those who God will connect to him in the future.

During his time of concertation, God allowed Apostle Brodnax to daily generate a devotional that highlighted key aspects that God wanted to speak on; key aspects that God wanted to release here in the earth realm. So, for forty-nine days Apostle not only fasted and prayed but he yielded all of him, to the will of God, to produce a prophetic devotional for healing of the mind, body, and soul. It is my prayer that you will allow the words written in this book the opportunity to cultivate healing in you. It has been my personal experience of witnessing these words to unfold right before my eyes. I applied these forty-nine days of devotion to my life and the pain that once attempted to consume my body had to be casted down and returned to its sender. I am healed.

~Prophetess Tykese Brodnax~

Prophetic Forecast

What are we seeing? What is Holy Spirit saying: We are seeing a cleansing of the Bride.

This is a time of purification for the Church. God is allowing the church to go through her purification while she is espoused. The wedding is closer than we think. I saw the words "Detachment".

We are in a time where God is causing leaders to fall back in love with their first love their families. So many Pastors and leaders have fell in love with Christ's Bride because of what she could provide for them.

This detachment is also a tool to set things back in order and cast out the spirit of adultery that has hit the church. Beware thou adulterous leaders who have taken the Bride and hid her in Your houses. I saw "49".

As the body of Christ, we need to find ourselves fasting and praying within the next 7 weeks. This is to prepare us for the last leg of the 7 months of purification of the bride that started in February. This will give us true insight for what lies ahead. September will be a change of tide and the roadmap to navigate through upcoming events will only be released in the spirit through denying your flesh.

Day 1: Realign us

God has you in a place where he is fine tuning you. Prepare to be re-invited to a deeper place

in God. While on your journey God is redefining purpose, redirecting destiny, and realigning

relationships. Enjoy this re-moment for this is a defining moment for your life.

Day 1

Healing shall take place in this area...

Day 2: Cleanse us Lord

So many times, we have plans and we expect the weather to be a certain way for our activities we planned. The Bible says there is a way that seems right to us but in the end, it may be foiled or destroyed. Have you ever felt your plans were ruined by rain? You picked the best day to plan your event or to do a certain thing and you wanted it to be right. This morning I got up as usual and started my day, hopped in the car, pulled out of the garage, the weather was nice, and it had a good breeze blowing. It reminded me of fall time, and I thanked God for the beautiful morning.

As I started down the street it begins to rain. Wait a minute the weather was exactly right, the breeze was right, and I got hit with rain and thought well this just messed the day up. As I got to work Holy Spirit took me to Ephesians where the word said: so that He might sanctify her, having cleansed her by the washing of water with the word, Then it hit me. My plans could have been different from what the will of the Father was. Therefore, he sent the rain/ water to do what the sea does to sandcastles at the beach. Wash it out so that we can rebuild another one or way. The Lord is trying to sanctify - set us apart by the water of his word. Today let the water of the word do the work to set you apart and bring about a much better day. Just know that even though it's rain, it's cleansing our thoughts and plans to make room for his will. Be blessed.

Day 2

Healing shall take place in this area...

Day 3: Find Rest

As we deal with the everyday hustle and bustle of life it is important that we find a place and space to sometimes do nothing. Science and Doctors say it is important for us to at least get 8 hours of sleep. This allows the body to rejuvenate, cells to repair, and ultimately take your mind off everything else.

Dr.'s also says if you don't get proper sleep that eventually your body will collapse and rest on its own. Sleeping gives you rest, peace and quiet, and your body the ability to rebuild itself.

I think on the spiritual side of things we need this type of rest also. Sometimes our spirit gets so noisy, busy, and over exerted that we begin to come unglued and ultimately collapse of spiritual fatigue. Sad to say many of us are so busy doing us and being in control of everything that we don't know how to rest.

Today I want to challenge you to find rest wherever you are no matter what you're up against. Jesus says take his yoke upon you rather he is saying give me yours and you take mine. For he is saying what I must deal with is easier. If you take my yoke you also get my faith, and my peace.

He says for I am gentle and humble. Jesus is basically saying throughout it all I make the calm. Jesus says then you will find rest for the part of you that need rest the most your soul and spirit.

Find your rest in Christ today. #Trade yours for his. For he says I give you peace not like the world gives but a peace only God can give that will allow you to rest even during a storm. Relax in him.

Day 3

Healing shall take place in this area...

Day 4: The wedge works

Today 6 weeks after my accident. 4 weeks after my surgery, 2 weeks of being off my feet, and 2 weeks of walking in a boot with 2 wedges in it. I am finally able to take 1 of the wedges out and my leg feels somewhat like it's getting back to normal.

As I was taking the wedges out, I begin to think why I had the wedges in the first place. The Surgeon gave me a recovery plan to get back to where I was before the accident. I begin to take notes. I think we all as believers can attest that sometimes even if we try to avoid them, we have accidents (sin, fall short). These accidents cripple us and halt us from doing what we normally do.

Can I suggest to you that our Surgeon (Jesus) has a recovery plan for us to get better, it may hurt a little bit, but sometimes all you need is a wedge. Something that stays between you and the part of you that was damaged in the accident. Maybe it's your mind, body, or soul. Maybe it's the fact that you feel you let God down by falling short after all you've done to avoid accidents. May I suggest to you that you can recover. You just need to use the wedge. Something that will stay between you and the damaged part.

Your wedge is repentance and the word. Apply these to the affected area and go on your way to be fully who you were pre-accident. Some look at a wedge as restrictions but really, it's restoration. A wedge says I know I'm not ready to handle the load of this right now because the damaged part is not strong enough yet. Today repent and apply the word so that you can heal. #wedgesworks

Day 4

Healing shall take place in this area...

Day 5: Find it.

Today I believe most of us will get up this Saturday morning and think what we are going to do today. Where can we go and what can we get done that we were not able to get done all week.

I suggest today you look for something that you probably had not had all week and that is peace. The Bible says that God created the earth and all that came with it in 6 days but on the 7th day he rested. Yes, God created a place and space for rest. Not because he was tired but rather because he understood that at some point in our journey, we need to take a rest.

And in that rest, we should find a peace. A peace that does nothing, owes nothing, and plans nothing. Peace that surpasses all understanding. Jesus told us that he gives us peace but not as the world gives us, but true peace so that we can rest when everything else is going crazy around us.

Yes, it's a pandemic and while others are looking for sanitizers, mask, and everything else that has them on the edge. I advise you to look for peace and when you find her do nothing. Happy Sabbath.

Day 5

Healing shall take place in this area...

Day 6: Understanding when the assignment has changed.

Many times, throughout our journey as a believer we get comfortable in our day to day processes and walk. We must be tuned to the heart of God to understand the frequency of what the spirit is calling for.

Not only does he call and justify he also assigns. You should never get complacent in where you are in Christ. Whenever you get comfortable it's a given that the assignment will change. God will use the seeds you've sown to usher you into your new assignment. Get ready for greatness in God. People walking away, appetite change, and confirmations are key indicators your assignment has changed.

Day 6

Healing shall take place in this area...

Day 7: Master it.

From the day we were born we begin to master things. We rely on the people and things around us to help us learn. After we learn them, we practice those things till we master them. It is only after we master them that we are truly ready for the next thing to master.

A person who never masters things is a person with many open doors in their mind and eventually their soul. As a child you must master milk before meat, crawl before walk, and potty before toilet. That is how it is in our spiritual life.

Most of us are ready for the next and we have never mastered the now. We are ready for a new position and we never mastered the now. Ready for a new spouse but we've never truly mastered loving the one we have now and never truly forgave anyone.

There is so much brokenness, anger, and emptiness when we don't master forgiving others. We have people tied to our very own curses of bad wishing, bitterness, and anger when we don't forgive. Truth of the matter we tie ourselves to the curse of unforgiveness and stagnate our own growth because not being able to forgive locks you in a box with the corporate and replays the incident over and over.

I truly admonish you today if you're ready to subdue (master) and have true dominion over everything in your life. First master the art of forgiveness. This unchains you, releases others, closes doors, and patch the holes in your soul that the enemy tries to anchor down in. Master forgiving today. Not I forgive but I want to forget. True forgiveness is like saying you slapped me last time, but I don't have guards up in case you want to slap me again. True forgiveness opens you up to forgive and receive. #Master it.

Day 7

Healing shall take place in this area...

Day 8: Make me new

Truth is we are drawn to that which we have gotten accustomed to. These things become a natural part of us, and we do them without knowing or thinking. Just like most of us David was drawn to and did things that had become second nature to him. David lived in rejection. He and his father's relationship wasn't the best. And because of this David had issues with relationships.

He never understood how to love. His perception of love was based off his relationship that he had with the sheep he spent most of his time with. It was based off protection not connection, and it was based off doing what he felt necessary to protect that which he had grown to love. Protection of what he spent most of his time with.

As we look at David, we see that this works well with sheep and not well with humans. David soon finds out the behavior he learned caused him to fail. He begins to ask God to forgive and help him but reminded God of how he was raised. We need to do a self-evaluation often to see what behavior we have practiced that has become part of us and is causing us to err. There comes a time we must call it out and put it on the table and ask God to purge and wash us so that we can tear down these strongholds in our life. After all what work for the animals doesn't always work for humans. So today ask God to create in us a new slate and renew the right spirit in us. Make me new.

Day 8

Healing shall take place in this area...

Day 9: Never alone

There is a story about this 5-year-old boy who is at the store with his mom. She is shopping and he is playing in the racks while she is shopping. Well mom moved a couple racks down and the boy never noticed he is just having the time of his life playing in racks. Mom moves an aisle over and thinks the boy moved with her, but he is having fun in the racks. However, 10 min pass and the boy notices that mom has moved, and he cannot find her. The boy starts crying and a stranger ask what is wrong and the boy said my mom left me.

The stranger takes the boy to the counter, they call for mom on the intercom, and mom shows up while the boy is still crying. The mom tells the boy to stop crying I never left you just got so caught up playing in the racks that you didn't move when I moved, but I knew where you were.

That is just like when some of us feel that God has abandoned us but truth of the matter, we got so caught up in playing that God moved and we did not. The focus of the story is the whole time Mom knew where he was. Just like mom God always knows where we are, he just waits for us to call out to him. Today we cast down fear and pray against the thoughts and spirit of abandonment that have crept into our lives as we got caught up. Today I declare you are found and free in the matchless name of Jesus.

Day 9

Healing shall take place in this area...

Day 10: He restores my soul....

Victorian Homes are sought after in the housing market because of the detail in architecture. These homes could be worth up to millions. The original builders put so much time and detail in planning and designing these homes that people still marvel at their beauty even now. Now even though these homes are sometimes hundreds of years old and need extensive repairs the owners never tear them down and rebuild they just restore. That is just like us I and God. These souls of ours were made with so much in mind and so much detail.

But after a while, after life, after our Will has had its way with the soul, we begin to have wear and tear. Holes pop up, soul ties get attached, and sometime the very foundation of our soul feels like it has shifted, but there is hope. Jesus is the architect that is waiting to do something with your soul. Seeing the condition of it he does not want to tear it down. After all there are some parts that makes this soul stand out that is different from the others. There are also some changes, and things that have happened to the soul that may be good after a few minor things have been restored.

So, our architect (Jesus) decides that instead of tearing it down he is going to restore it. He restores our soul. The restoration process does not just bring it back to its original look and purpose, but it also adds more value. Today I suggest we all let him do what he wants to do. Restore us, make us better, and repair the broken parts. Today may restoration be your portion in every area of your life.

Day 10

Healing shall take place in this area...

Day 11: Live

When I passed by you and saw you squirming in your blood, I said to you while you were in your blood, 'Live!' Yes, I said to you while you were in your blood, 'Live" (Ezekiel 16:6)! Today like God told us in Ezekiel I am commanding you to "Live". As you read this passage you would read that God say I saw you in a pool of blood. Nobody washed you off after you were born. Nobody cut your cord. It is like you were born and people just left you live in a field.

Truth of the matter we feel that way sometimes. After going through something and we see the mess that we are in. Many of us just lay there and spiritually die. But God say no so. Another way to look at it is this child is just in the middle of nowhere existing. Not living, not moving, no goals, no aspirations, just there. It is a shame that most of us are just like this child just existing.

Today I ask you to look at where you are. Though all this mess is around you. Though you have made a mess of things. Though life and relationships have hurt you and left you just existing. I command you to live and come forth just like Lazarus, just like the Damsel Jesus raised, just like the shunamite's son. God is saying I saw you, but I am saying live. Family it is time to live again, love again, and laugh again. Get up!!

Day 11

Healing shall take place in this area...

Day 12: Special delivery

Psalms 120: 20

He sent His word and healed them and delivered them from their destructions. Isn't that

something. At FedEx or UPS, you can ship packages across the world. They guarantee the

package will be there with-in three days for ground shipments. However, if you want to

ensure your package gets there at a certain time you pay for special delivery.

This could be overnighted, Saturday Delivery, 1st day or 2nd day Air. The purpose

is to get it there when you need it. Basically, you pay more to get more. It comes with a

surety. I want to let you know on this Sabbath that God paid more to get more, and it comes

with a special delivery. In Psalms 120 starting at verse 17 we read how fools (one that

despised wisdom and say there is no God) had set themselves up for destruction. Isn't that

something we mess things up our selves. We find ourselves at the point of death, we cry out

to God, he is so merciful, that at the point of destruction, right before we check out, he moves.

He sends help and a special delivery. His word. The Bible says he sent his word and

it healed us and delivered us from our destruction. The things that were going to happen were

ours, we owned and earned it. But he sent his word to heal and deliver us. Meaning he healed

us and moved us out of the way of self-inflicted death and destruction. Today let us be

thankful for his loving kindness and tender mercies. Receive your healing and deliverance

today because they go together. Happy Sabbath.

Day 12

Healing shall take place in this area...

Day 13: Rise Up

Imagine the hustle and bustle of the day at a pool of Jesus' time. Everyone is eager and excited to see what is going to happen next when these angels trouble the water. Who will be healed, who will be delivered, who would be set free?

Suddenly Jesus walks into this community pool and ask a man. Do you want to be well? Already knowing that he had been in that position for a longtime he yet asks him. Do you want to be well?

The reason I believe he ask is that some of us have been in a situation so long that we do not have the faith to be healed or free. The man instead of saying yes gives him an excuse of why he is not healed already.

As if he (the impotent man) was saying do you think I just want to be here, or I have not tried to help myself. Jesus basically ignores the explanation and excuses and says, "Rise up".

Today I want to tell you your excuses and explanation of why not do not even matter it is time for you to go. Rise up in Jesus name. Tell the people around you today "Don't be surprised when you see me rise".

Day 13

Healing shall take place in this area…

Day 14: Turn it over

Mark Chapter 11:15 Jesus walks into the temple and without question or explanatio drives people and things that did not belong out and overturned the tables. To drives means he forcibly put into motion these things. You must understand that he drove the things and people that did not belong and overturned these tables. Tables represent commonality, communion, and invitation. So many of us have welcomed things in our spirits and souls tha did not belong and invited these things to the table. They have seats and they are thieves as Jesus calls them. They are selling off our peace, joy, and happiness. Sad thing is most of us have invited them. So today it is time for you to take possession of your temple, drive them out, and overturn the tables. Your body is the temple of the Holy Ghost. Let us cleanse it today.

Day 14

Healing shall take place in this area...

Day 15: Lord heal our land

Imagine this: the souls and spirits of man can become so corrupt that it begins to corrupt everything around him. I believe that we are living in such a time. You ever noticed that pollution not only affects that site at which it was released but it spreads. People our sins are just like pollution. When we allow ourselves to be engulfed by these evils it will surely affect everything around us even the land.

The Bible says the wicked shall be turned into hell, and all the nations that reject God. We need the Lord in every part of our lives but when we reject him out of our personal space, we also reject him and eject him out of our land. Surely, we can't move God out, but our rejection and sin moves his hand, his healing, and his protection. Eventually our whole land is filled with sin and shame. Our houses, businesses, and churches need a cleansing. Lord purge us that we shall be clean, wash us that we can be whiter that snow. We cry out to you for our land needs a healing. Our community needs healing, our nation needs healing.

Lord we know you called us, today we humbly submit to your will, we repent, we pray, we seek you, and not your hand. We ask that you move upon us and begin to heal this land. We are talking about us. Heal us so we can be a source of strength and healing for someone else. Lord today heal the land(me).

Day 15

Healing shall take place in this area...

Day 16: From barren to bountiful

As I was awakening this morning, I heard the words "Produce after its kind". That is, it! We were put here on earth to do more than exist. Every living thing God created he gave the commandment to "produce after its kind".   Though the commandment is released many of us are still barren. Not just in the physical but spiritually also. To be barren means that land or place is too poor to produce much of anything. Most of us are too poor in the spirit to reproduce after ourselves. Jesus says blessed are the poor in spirit for theirs is the kingdom of heaven. But this is for those that say I know heaven is mine, but I want to produce in the earth.

Whether it is naturally or spiritually God gave the command for things to produce after its kind and we are about to go from barren to bountiful. I command everything around you to be fruitful and multiply and subdue. Today take control of your thoughts, subdue those negative stigmas you have put on yourself it's time to be fruitful. We decree we are about to go from barren to bountiful in Jesus name.

Day 16

Healing shall take place in this area...

Day 17: Touch what is touching him

Sometimes we feel so far away. So, pressed. So sick in our condition that we cannot see a way out nor a way through. We are in a place where we cannot see how we can get to Jesus with all that's going on with us and in us. I'm reminded of the woman with the issue of blood who was just like that. Who couldn't be seen in public because of her condition.   It's funny how we can be going through something and feel just like her. We feel our condition will not let us see him.

I suggest today that if you're down, wrapped up, tied up, and tangled up in something that will not allow you to see him face to face; just touch what's touching him. Perhaps you just don't feel worthy; just touch what's touching him. I suggest if you feel like you are not worthy enough, healthy enough, or strong enough to see him just touch what's touching him. It may be a person that's touching him. A ministry that's touching him. A television program that's touching him. Get close enough to what's touching him.

The woman with the issue of blood said if I can just touch the hem of him, I shall be made whole. Today let's touch the hem of him and watch this blood dry up. It took all that she had to give it all to him.

#touch what's touching him.

Day 17

Healing shall take place in this area...

Day 18: Put it out there!

People tend to hide when there is something wrong with them. The reason being is that we as people like to look perfect in the eyes of others even if it's just make believe. We don't like negative attention or the feeling of being less of.

I'm reminded today of the man Jesus healed with the withered hand. I imagine he was just like one of us from the wrist up we look normal but the wrist down everyone can see something is wrong. I imagine he spent most of the time hiding his withered hand so he wouldn't get negative attention.

Can I suggest to you that hiding doesn't get you healed. I always say you can't get help hiding. At some point we must understand that we can only heal what's been revealed. So, this man is in front of Jesus and as Jesus said one thing "Stretch forth your hand". I t's like he was saying instead of hiding that hand "Put it out there" stretch forth that hand, show it.

You can read the story and find out as soon as he put it out there it was healed. Today I only have one message to get you closer to your healing. "Put it out there" whatever that's damaged , broken, or just need healing. #Put it out there

Day 18

Healing shall take place in this area...

Day 19: A call for help

LORD my God, I called to you for help, and you healed me." — Psalm 30:2 You want healing? Then you must want help. The Psalmist lets us know that we can get healing without saying a word about it. He tells us that he called for help and the Lord healed. That is amazing. A simple call or cry for help brings on healing. This shows us that some of the things we need help with (relationships, mental anguish, etc) may be things we need to be healed from. Yesterday we said put it out there today we say call it out. Call on the Lord so your healing can take place. Shalom....

Day 19

Healing shall take place in this area...

Day 20: Let God do what God do....

And the prayer of faith shall save the sick, and the Lord shall raise him up; and if he has committed sins, they shall have forgiven him (James 5:15).

The scriptures say the prayer of faith shall save the sick and the Lord shall raise him up. Looking at this scripture and what caught my attention is the prayer of faith shall save the sick. The writer tells us that if we are sick call for the elders, let them anoint us, and pray. It says that this prayer is going to save us. I believe the writer is expressing to us that prayer will help save us from worry, doubt, and anxiety over what's ailing us.

But ultimately it is God who is going to do the major healing. Too often we put our emphasis of the point of man praying when praying of me is just part of the healing process. We should be waiting on the raising of God. The Bible says we can pray but it's God that will raise us up. Happy Sunday saints give it all to God today. Shalom...

Day 20

Healing shall take place in this area...

Day 21: He got this!

Fear thou not; for I am with thee be not dismayed; for I am thy God (Psalms 41:10). Often fear becomes the main corporate to attribute to our lack of faith and trust in God. We read the scriptures, we hear the testimonies, but one bad prognosis can send all of what we've seen and heard out the window. The scriptures, testimonies, and what we see are pillars of our faith these are what got us here. Today I want you to think on what you've seen God do, and heard God do. And once you get these in your mind do not let go.

This is your antidote to the fear that comes along with whatever you're facing. God told the Psalmist in the A part of this scripture: Fear not and the reason you don't have to fear follows directly behind it "for I am with thee". Today know that the Lord is with you no matter what you face. And be not dismayed for he is God. Did you forget that he is God? He got this!!!!

Day 21

Healing shall take place in this area...

Day 22: Get ready to smile and tell it!!

One interpretation of the word Miracle in the Greek is miraculom interpreted as an object of wonder. Today I want you to get ready to smile because you are about to see a wonder. God is releasing a flow from the healing fountains of heaven that runs from under his throne. Oh yes there is a river, there is healing, and there is a miracle released with you in mind. Whatsoever it may be. Healing for your body, your heart, or your soul. Get ready you're about to be in awe in the next 26 days. Get ready to tell somebody and publish his wonderous work!!!! That I may publish with the voice of thanksgiving, and tell of all thy wondrous works (Psalms 26:7)

Day 22

Healing shall take place in this area...

Day 23: The secret place for the seekers

There is a place where healing and deliverance meet the hurting and depressed. I know we have so many places where we go to get what we need. The grocery store for groceries, the pharmacy for medicines, and the gym for exercise.

I want to introduce you to a place where those that have been praying and waiting o God to do something can dwell while waiting. This is the secret place. Where you can let your hair down, drop your guards and be vulnerable before your God. The place where you and him meet. The place where there's a private practice operating in all sorts of healing and deliverance. This is the place for "the generation" that will seek him.

The generation that will seek and look for him to the point that they begin to dwell there and once there life is renewed, joy is unleashed, and healing is plentiful as the pine needles on a heathy pine tree. I encourage you to join the generation and get all you need. For Psalms 24:6 says: This is the generation of them that seek him, that seek thy face, O Jacob. Selah.

Day 23

Healing shall take place in this area...

Day 24: Leave my peace alone

There is a law against disturbing the peace. Whereby one could be convicted and sentenced for doing such an act. It's amazing that in the world there is such a law, but as we come into Christiandom we don't hold such a law, but we should. The reason being is that Jesus told us that he gives us peace but not as the world gives it. So, the world gives peace, and makes a law concerning the peace that it has allowed. The world subsequently has the right to enforce it's law and uphold it.

Can I suggest to you that in Christ we have the same ability as it relates to our peace. Why? Because the chastisement of our peace was upon him. Meaning the rebuke, criticism, or the reprimand of our peace was put in his possession. Therefore, everything that comes for our peace is added to his caseload and he handles it so we can have peace. Christ rebukes the disturbers of our peace. To sum it up give all the problems to Jesus and you hold on to the peace. For he was wounded for our transgressions, bruised for our iniquities, the chastisement of our peace was upon him, and by his stripes we are healed (Isaiah 53:5).

Day 24

Healing shall take place in this area...

Day 25: FaceTime

FaceTime has become an extremely popular application and feature to all expensive iPhone. It allows the user to get in contact with the receiver by not just talking to them but seeing them at the same time. The thing that makes this even more interesting is that to use FaceTime both parties must have the same phone type. They must both be on the same operating system. This is just as it is when it comes to the healing power of Jesus. Sometimes all we need is to be on the same operating system (faith). The faith operating system gives us the opportunity to have FaceTime with the master and get all that we need.

Today I suggest you upgrade your system and get a little FaceTime in. Your healing is nigh. Get ready to publish what Christ has done. Go show yourself to the priest. And it came to pass, when he was in a certain city, behold a man full of leprosy: who seeing Jesus fell on his face, and besought him, saying, Lord, if thou wilt, thou canst make me clean (Luke 5:12). And he put forth his hand, and touched him, saying, I will: be thou clean. And immediately the leprosy departed from him.

Day 25

Healing shall take place in this area…

Day 26: Double dose it

Today I pray you have a supernatural double dose of happiness to invade your very existence. Too often are we too serious, too worried, and too stressed. We are in this state to the point that a broken spirit takes over and eventually consumes us. The Proverb says: A merry heart doeth good like a medicine:
but a broken spirit drieth the bones.

Basically, it's saying being happy may not cure the issue, but it gives you relief. Not all medicines cure but they do help to relieve the pain and symptoms of the underlying ailment (the heart). I believe we need this to keep our spirits from drying out. The Psalmist says as the deer pants for the water so does my spirit pant for you God in a dry and thirsty land (Psalm 42:1). We must be careful to not let our hearts get so sick that it begins to flow into our spirit and begin to cause a drought. Today live, love, and laugh. Take your medicine, be merry, and watch your outlook change. Take a double dose of happiness.

Day 26

Healing shall take place in this area...

Day 27: They forget but I won't....

Too many times do we do things out of the kindness of our hearts. We do these things to help those that are less fortunate, bring closure to those that are open from past hurts, and to do our due diligence as being the hands and feet of God. The love of God and God's people are our reasons. Not for fame nor notoriety, not for clout, or even a reward. We do it because Holy Spirit leads us and it's our Christian duty.

I want to encourage you, whom just like me has helped to push and encourage others to know that God sees, and he knows. While others forget your acts of charity, and your love just know God says I see, and I remember. Isaiah 49:16, God lets us know that he knows, and he cares so much that he has inscribed us in the Palm of his hands. That is right your name is tattooed on the palm of the mighty hand of God. He then says your walls are ever before more. He's not talking about your room or you house but the walls of your heart. Because everything that you've done out of love was from the heart. Be encouraged to know others may forget but God won't.... Blessings.

Day 27

Healing shall take place in this area...

Day 28: You're getting stronger!

Job 17:9 The righteous also shall hold on his way, and he that hath clean hands shall be stronger and stronger. Get up! Wash your face! Wash your Faith! and put on your track suit. I declare you are getting stronger and stronger.

Job says the righteous shall hold their own. Meaning there is nothing that can move or beset you. Oh! but those who have clean hands and righteousness together shall get stronger and stronger.

Stronger in your faith. Stronger in your walk. I can see you in the spirit putting on spiritual muscle. It's like you're getting ready for a championship bout. And while the devil is getting tired and tired every round, you're getting stronger and stronger. I speak healing to your spirit and command you to stretch, you're about to get stronger and stronger.

Day 28

Healing shall take place in this area...

Day 29: Get your power back

Have you ever been under the influence of something? Meaning you are doing things that you know you shouldn't do, but it's out of your control. It's like your body is a car and something or someone else is driving it to do things that you know you shouldn't do. As God heals us, he wants to pull back layer after layer. He wants to deal with the thing's others can see. He wants to heal the places that already look healed. He wants to deliver us right now.

I was reading a scripture where the Apostle Paul says everything may be lawful but not expedient meaning - it may be a right thing but not the right time. Or it simply means just because you can does not mean you should. Many of us do things because we can and before you know it that thing is causing us to do it now because it wills. That's right that very thing has taken over your will, now it has taken over, it wills the things you do.

This is addiction. Jesus never meant for us to be ruled by anything except Holy Spirit and if we are, this is not the will of God concerning us. Today our prayer is that you lay these addictions out in front of the most High. The Bible says there is no temptation that are not common to man, but the Lord also has created ways to escape. It's time to escape the clutches of this thing once and for ever. Today we pray Lord forgive us for our sins, and cleanse us from unrighteousness. Lord we denounce ______________(addiction) and ask you to deliver us. Take away the taste and desire and give us peace and strength. Lord give us back our dominion over addiction(s) in Jesus name. Dominate and demonstrate saints. All things are lawful for me," but not all things are helpful. "All things are lawful for me," but I will not be dominated by anything (1 Cor.6:12).

Day 29

Healing shall take place in this area...

Day 30: He sees. He hears. He knows..

The Bible says the Lords eyes are over the righteous, and his ears are open to their prayers. So, whether we know it or not our God is all his majesty, in all that he could be doing, is watching over us.

God created all and he watches over it all but know for sure his eyes are over the righteous. Being righteous gives us the assurance that God sees. When people hurt us, wrong us, use us, or treat us right God sees.

Also, when we cry out to him about our many situations whether he says anything he hears everything. Every hurtful word, every thought that is spoken in our mind about our self he hears. Many us of cry out in our soul, or the mind of our spirit. We are depressed, confused, and may think low of ourselves because of past failures and misfortunes. I want to encourage you today that God sees, God hears, and he knows. Rest assured today that he is right there, and your help is too.

Day 30

Healing shall take place in this area...

Day 31: Let Jesus have it

Is. 53:4 Says "Surely" he has borne our griefs and carried our sorrows. This grief in Hebrew means sicknesses. Surely, he has borne(embodied) our sicknesses and carried away everything that has troubled us and caused us sadness.

I am so glad to know today that whatever ails me had already been intercepted in Christ. That means I need to understand that I don't have to deal with any ailments or sorrow. Why? Because Jesus took care of those two things for me.

Surely means without question, without doubt. It means that whatever comes after that "Surely" is absolute. I want us to know without a doubt today Jesus takes on our sickness and carries away our worry. So today let him have it so you can live your best life. Let go and let God!

Day 31

Healing shall take place in this area...

Day 32: The strength of your spirit

Proverbs 18:14 says......The spirit of a man will sustain his infirmity;

but a wounded spirit who can bear?

I suggest today we check on the health of our spirit. For it is our spirit that can keep us going even if we have sickness in our body. If we have sickness in our body a strong spirit will make sure we don't have sickness in our mind(infirmity).

Infirmity is when the sickness in your body has got to your mind. Therefore, we need often to do a spiritual and faith check up to make sure our spirit hasn't been wounded(breached). If the enemy or life breaches and wounds our spirit, it's only a matter of time before what is natural begins to seep into the spiritual and cause damage in our mind.

You are stronger than you think. Cancer can't rule, diabetes can't stay, and any other ailment will not take you down as long as you have a strong spirit. The Bible has never lied nor has it ever steered us wrong. I ask you to embody this principal about your spirit that says "The spirit of a man will keep him alive and living instead of just existing if it is strong. Today check your spirit.

Day 32

Healing shall take place in this area...

Day 33: Run in....

Proverbs says the name of the Lord is a strong tower. Can you imagine that? So much power in the name alone. Some trust in horses, some in chariots but we can trust in the name. The name of God alone is enough to save, heal, protect, and deliver. So many times, we wait for a move of God not realizing the power in the name. The name of the Lord is a strong tower, the righteous runneth into it and are saved. Get in the name!!!! Better yet run into it!!

Day 33

Healing shall take place in this area…

Day 34: He's keeping it together

Which holdeth our soul in life, and suffereth not our feet to be moved. You need to thank God for all that he does. He keeps it all together. The Psalmist says God's name is to be praised because he holds our soul in life. Think about like this without God your soul would slip right out of your body. He is the spiritual magnet needed to keep us all together. Though things may be falling apart around you it's ok to thank God for he holds your soul in life.

Day 34

Healing shall take place in this area...

Day 35: The wealthy place

If we were to all do a mental and spiritual inventory. Chances are we will be amazed at how far we have come. Amazed at the trials we had come through. Amazed at the fact we are still standing in our right mind, with a good heart.

That's right we could be bitter but we're not. We could be angry, but by the grace of God we're not. Truth is it's like we have been tried in the fire, drugged through the waters but we are still here, still standing, and still believing God.

And because we didn't give up and throw in the towel we are in a different place. A different demographic in the spirit. Truth is God never lets us go through things to come out the same. If we go through, we are coming out better. In a better mindset, better spiritually. We're in another place. The place where John said that I would that you would prosper and be in health even as your souls prosper. This place is the wealthy place where prosperity is on every facet of your life and being. Today rejoice, shout, and find your praise because God has caused men to ride over our heads; we went through fire and through water: but thou (God) brought us out into a wealthy place.

Day 35

Healing shall take place in this area...

Day 36: There is a healing flow

As I was sitting and reading Psalms this morning, I ran across the passage that said we were fearfully and wonderfully made) Psalm 139:14). That means we were not just thrown together, but rather God himself took time and patience to create us.

Every detail down to our eyelashes to toenails were carefully planned and engineered. How dare sickness and disease have any part of us if God didn't design us with it? Oh, but there is a flow of healing released today.

I heard the Lord say repent and be healed. It's just that simple repent your healing is waiting. The flow is released the rivers are open, but repentance is your admission.

Day 36

Healing shall take place in this area...

Day 37: He is big enough

To magnify something is to take and look at the said thing under a special lens. This lens magnifies or make the object look bigger than what it is. It allows the viewer to see more detail and get a better focus on the said object no matter how small it is.

I've noticed in my life I have magnified the wrong things at times. Not that I necessarily used a physical magnification lens but a mental one. I admit at times in my mind I made things that were small, big.

So many little arguments turned into big fights. Small mistakes had big consequences and it was linked to how I looked at the situation. I guess I made a few things bigger than what they should've been.

To think of it now, I even allowed small things to be bigger than God In my mind. Like a bad Dr.'s report, trouble in relationships, financial troubles, and just life.

This morning the Psalmist said my soul shall make her boast in the Lord meaning she has a right to be big, to be seen, to be proud, and it's all because she (my soul) is in the Lord (Psalm 34:2). Where protection, direction, and peace are.

And those that are humble just as I have been will be glad for me. Understanding I am because of him and I do because of him. But what gets me is immediately after celebrating us or himself the Psalmist says that's cool but let's magnify the Lord.

Let's look at God through a different lens in the spirit. He is already a big God we cannot make him any bigger, but we can begin to look at the detail. How that he steps in right on time, heals with a blink of an eye, love through the passion of Christ, and sets us free.

Today let's magnify God and exalt his name forever.

Day 37

Healing shall take place in this area...

Day 38: Find that rest

To many times we are too busy to stop and reflect. The Lord in his infinite wisdom saw that rest would be a necessity for us therefore in all his creating he created a day to rest. That's right, a whole 24-hour calendar day to do nothing but relax, reflect, and rest.

This sabbath was created with us in mind. Knowing that one day life, work, family, and being fruitful would tire us out. Most ailments in the body can be fought off with rest.

Resting from eating (fasting) brings about healing. Resting from being awake (sleeping) causes the body to go into repair mode and rejuvenate itself.

Today let's focus on a new rest. Resting in the Lord. To rest in the Lord means I relinquish all rights and privileges to my troubles and desires and give them to the lord. Trut is; if we are honest most of the stuff that's troubling us is too big for us anyway.

So why not rest in him. The Psalmist says: Rest in the LORD and wait patiently for him (Psalm 37:7).

So today as we are on this journey together let's have a mental sabbath and rest in the Lord.

Day 38

Healing shall take place in this area...

Day 39: The face of hope

Psalms 39:6 Surely every man walketh in a vain shew: surely, they are disquieted in vain:
he heapeth up riches, and knoweth not who shall gather them.

Basically, saying that we walk in vain meaning we try to present this high standard or do
things to get people to receive us as such. Truth of the matter just as much as we are trying to
prove we are still pitiful on the inside.

So, we build this life, gather these things just so people can look at us and see success.
Really, we spend most of our life trying to keep up with the Jones's. This behavior is so
unhealthy and will cause infirmity because it's never enough.

Once you build this image the stress comes when you must maintain, and failure is inevitable.
I like the Psalmist in this chapter because he quickly focuses his attention on God.

He says people do this in vain, they heap up riches not knowing who will inherit it. The
Psalmist says while they are doing this. What are we waiting for, but oh Lord our hope is in
you.

Instead of racking your brain to impress others today. Let's wait on God to do what he wants
to do. Put your hope in him and watch the outcome. Faith in God is the face of hope.

Day 39

Healing shall take place in this area...

Day 40: He anoints my head

Today our thanksgiving should be based solely on the love God has for us. It surpasses our brittle intellect, confuses our rationale, and conveys his love in strength and power. It's strong love. It's powerful love. It's a love we have never known before or could even fathom. Not obsessive, not possessive, but pure love. The type of love that does and wants anything in return. Like: I'll wake you up and expect nothing in return. The type of love like I shield and protect you and you owe me nothing. The type of love like I will anoint your head. To many it may be nothing. Except when God anoints your head it's not just to pour oil or to smear.

This anointing of our head comes with intentional love, and intentional purpose. To the naked eye it's a kind jester to us it is protection. He anoints our head with oil. He is the great Sheep master. The good shepherd. When he anoints our head it's to protect us from the things we don't see. The shepherd anoints the sheep's head to keep parasites and bugs from infesting and killing the sheep. He anoints the head and the ears and smears it on purpose. To keep these deadly things out of the ears so that they can't nest in the ears and eventually reach the brain. You better thank God today because a lot of things that could've got in your brain through your ears but didn't because of his anointing. He anoints our head with oil. Now live in the green pastures prepared for you. #shabatshalom

Day 40

Healing shall take place in this area...

Day 41: To bind the broken hearted

Isaiah prophesied it. Jesus said it. The Spirit of the Lord GOD is upon me; because the LORD hath anointed me to preach good tidings unto the meek; he hath sent me to bind up the brokenhearted, to proclaim liberty to the captives (Isaiah 61:1).

That's right God has anointed us to preach the gospel to the poor and sent us to bind up the brokenhearted. Most people with broken hearts get reclusive and isolated. It's our job as the church to go to them.

We have been sanctioned by God to help gather those pieces that are broken and help pull it together so that they can begin to heal. Today we pray for every broken heart. That as we have been anointed and sent to them to bind those pieces and healing will begin.

Day 41

Healing shall take place in this area...

Day 42: The day of the double

What if I told you that everything that you went through is about to pay you? Yes, you're about to be paid for your humiliation, your shame, and your confusion. Today I declare you are about to move into "Double".

Double your healing, double your breakthrough, double your deliverance, double your finances. Yes, you worked through it. There was labor so there must be wages. Muzzle not the ox that treadeth the corn.

Get ready payday has arrived. Your address has been upgraded. Your land has a new name. I decree double for your trouble. For all that 20/20 has brought you shall receive double. Not 20 for 20 but 20 for 40. Watch God do it in Jesus name. If your receive this put #Double on your wall.

Is. 61:7

The year of the double. For your shame ye shall have double; and for confusion they shall rejoice in their portion: therefore, in their land they shall possess the double: everlasting joy shall be unto them.

Day 42

Healing shall take place in this area…

Day 43: Don't throw it away... there is a blessing in it.

As we regain ground and go about to establish our new level of healing, deliverance, and love. We need to be careful not to get rid of things that have a blessing in them.

The crazy thing is when going through we can never see the blessing. While in sickness we can never see the healing. While in relationship trouble we can never see the blessing.

We never see the blessings of things that cause heartache, struggle, tears, and discomfort due to the packaging and end up trying to throw away good stuff.

God tells Isaiah and his people in chapter 65:8a

Thus, saith the LORD, "as the new wine is found in the cluster, and one saith, Destroy it not; for a blessing is in it".

I want you to know your joy may be like new wine. Locked in a cluster of anything. Pain, hurt, humiliation, or struggle. Don't throw it away. I see so many people say just throw 2020 away. I hear God say, "Don't throw it away there's a blessing in it". There's healing in it, there peace in it, there's increase in it!

Day 43

Healing shall take place in this area…

Day 44: Don't forget the wounds!

Most of the time when we think of healing we only think of the ailment or the sickness. I think that we don't realize that even if we hadn't had surgery that's sickness sometimes leave a wound.

Maybe not a physical wound in all situations but if you've dealt with real sickness or infirmit there is always a wound. Rather in your spirit, body, or soul.

So, we get healed our health gets restored and we go on about our day to day never to do wound care. This open wound can set up infection and could be worse than the original pain Check the wounds!

I'm glad that God not only restores our health, but he also heals and treats the wounds that ar left behind and sometimes untreated. Wounds be healed today in Jesus name.

"'But I will restore you to health and heal your wounds,' declares the LORD…"(Jeremiah 30:17).

Day 44

Healing shall take place in this area...

Day 45: We always win

As we bring these days to a close, we need to always give honor where honor is due. After all we have come this far only by the grace of God. Many of us have endured hardship, health challenges, disappointments, trials, and tribulations, and at times we felt we were losing ground and our grip.

But thanks be to God that we are still here, still standing, still striving, and still smiling. Why because through it all we had the victory. It may have looked bad. Yes, it may have looked unfavorable. But thanks be to God who always causes us to win.

That's right we have help from on high and a reason to be thankful. For God always causes us to triumph. Meaning the race is staged, the fight is rigged and with the help of God we always win. Walk in your victory.

Day 45

Healing shall take place in this area...

Day 46: Strength and grace

The Psalmist says Honor and majesty are before him: strength and beauty are in his sanctuary (Psalm 96:6).

I want you to know as you are walking out your healing that God is walking it out with you. And where God is honor and majesty is there. That's right, right where you are the courts of heaven is evoking an angelic presence of praise and worship. This praise and worship are solely based on the honor and majesty of our Lord. He deserves all honor and praise for what he has done for us. Honor and majesty stand still in his presence.

So, while in his presence and your healing is manifesting make sure to get to the safe place. The place of refuge, the place of peace, and the place life. While others are running from and talking about the sanctuary. You better get there.

For in his sanctuary is strength and beauty. In his sanctuary is the power to come out and the grace to endure. Beauty is this Psalm is translated into grace. You better thank God today that even though you wouldn't have chosen to go through it and do it. He gave you the strength and grace to do it. May Strength and grace be your portion today.

Day 46

Healing shall take place in this area...

Day 47: Seasons change

Ecclesiastes says to everything under the Sun there are times and seasons. It amazes me we are accepting of that fact and scream it's a new season, but we are reluctant to change. Whether we understand it or not change is a season.

With it being difficult to explain and even the more difficult to understand. Change is complicated and a terror to the complacent. To many changes is all too unpleasant but it is necessary. As you embrace the new you with all that the Lord has done to heal you. It's time to embrace change and embrace it as a season of change.

I declare in your season of change your mind will change, your drive will change, your creativity will change and it is necessary to harness the new level of power and anoint being released in your season of change. Embrace it. It's a new season!

Day 47

Healing shall take place in this area…

Day 48: Live long

This Sunday I want to encourage you to live. Not just any kind of life. When the world tells you to live it means to be riotous, do whatever you want to do. After all they would say you only live once. Truth of the matter you only die physically once but today I want you to be encouraged. Because if you put your trust and faith in God allow him to lead and guide you. Allow God to heal every part of you that's wounded. You will live.

Not just any old life but a long full life. The Psalmist said with long life will God satisfy him. In Hebrew that word satisfy means to give it, to have in abundance. God is saying today I will give you that abundant life. The rest of the scripture says to show him my salvation. Meaning I'm going to give you long life or abundant life to show you what salvation does. Salvation doesn't just save you from hell and the lake. Salvation preserves your life. For our life is hid in his.

Day 48

Healing shall take place in this area...

Day 49: Take up your bed and take off!

As we close this journey out, I want to encourage you to prepare to take up your bed and take off. That's right take off. Take off that old mindset that you got accustomed to while you were down.

Take of that paralyzed talk that you developed while you were down. Take off those negative emotions and feelings you developed while you were down. This is not the time nor space for anything that will keep you confined to that old place.

The conversations, the eyes, the sidebars, and the spectators are about to be put to shame. Why? Because that same bed that they saw you bound to they are about to see you carrying. So today just as Jesus asked the man at the pool would he be made whole?

I am asking you. The man in the story gave an excuse of why he was not healed already by blaming others for wanting there healing more than him. Today Holy Spirit snatch your excuses and give you strength to say it's my turn.

You have seen everybody else get theirs, now it's time for you to get your just due. Take up your bed today and don't just walk, take off! You will stay healed, delivered, and set free. I decree perpetual healing to be released in every area of your life.

Day 49

Healing shall take place in this area...

9 798552 972470